Tai Chi: The Beginners Guide to Tai Chi Exercises, Moves, and Balancing Energy

Lori P.

Contents

What is Tai Chi?

Tai Chi is a low impact, weight bearing and aerobic, yet relaxing exercise which began as a martial art form.

As this martial art form developed, it gained the purpose of improving physical and mental health. Tai Chi is practiced in many styles, it involves slow, gentle movements, deep breathing and meditation. The form of meditation in Tai Chi is called moving meditation. Some even believe that Tai Chi improves the energy flow through your body, leading to awareness of yourself, a calm and overall sense of wellness. Staying healthy and physically fit does not mean you have to sacrifice your free hours in the gym doing heavy exercises and workouts along with dieting. You do not have to do strenuous workouts and maintain a diet to stay fit. There is a way you can maintain a good shape and maintain a healthy mind and physique and that is through Tai Chi. This can be done regardless of the location, status in the society and the age. Tai Chi is considered as a form of meditative healing technique for centuries and has soothing and calming effects. Tai Chi has many movements which are defined as an extremely low impact exercise which has a low impact on the muscles and joints which relieve you from stress.

With proper implementation of techniques and movements a great and desired effects of flexibility, function, strength, balance and relaxation can be obtained.

Tai Chi has a lot of benefits; it protects the elderly from risk of falls, high blood pressure, multiple sclerosis, chronic stroke etc. It protects the people from stress and induces relaxation. It is effective in reducing depression, stress and anxiety.

These are just a few benefits of Tai Chi. With its benefits and no side effects and easy to practice nature, it is safe and reasonable to practice this ancient form of exercising. Tai Chi promotes physical and mental health.

Tai Chi - A History

Tai Chi started as a martial art form but years down it is being down to improve the health, physically and mentally. Tai Chi was created in the 17th century. Tai Chi literally means great ultimate fist.

Tai Chi stems back to the times which are now shredded by legend. The early practitioners of Tai Chi understood that life and universe's other matter consists of energy and was born out by modern physics when Einstein proved that energy and matter is the same. The Chinese called this as Chi, others call this is as "ki" or "prana" which is a concept used in many healing arts.

If the Chi has to be healthy in the body, it has to be on the move constantly. A stagnant chi will lead to illness and disease. Tai Chi was developed to promote the movement of Chi through the human body.

Tai Chi Styles

Tai Chi styles are practiced in many schools which are practice all around the world. They are:

1. Chen
2. Yang
3. Wu Yu Chian
4. Wu Jian
5. Sun

Chen style

The Chen Style is the basis of all modern Tai Chi styles, it was developed by a family with the name Chen. They lived close to Shaolin temple and were known for their martial arts skill, but focuses on the development of the flow of Chi.

Yang

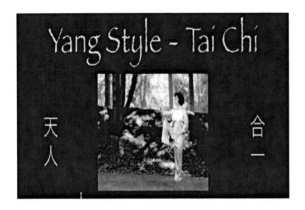

Another Shaolin Kung Fu martial artist, Yang Lu Chan undertook Tai Chi training from the Chen family. He studied the Chen style for many years and passed his skills to his surviving sons and grandson. This style of Tai Chi is the most popular form of Tai Chi.

Wu Yu Xian

The Yang and Chen styles of Tai Chi influenced the development of Wu Yu Xian style as the founder Wu Yu Xian originally trained with Yang Lu Chan and Chen Quing Ping. After years of training he developed a new style, using the elements of his masters. This form is not widely practices outside China.

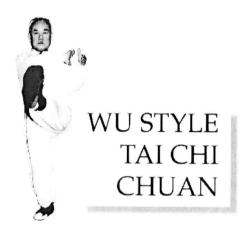

WU STYLE TAI CHI CHUAN

In the early 20th century, this style became popular in China. It is second popular form of Tai Chi which became popular across the globe.

Sun Style

This is the last style of Tai Chi. Like other styles, it is named after the family which developed this style, Sun Lu Tang. This is the newest of all the styles of Tai Chi and it grew from the sun training in many martial arts and the Wu Yu Xian style of Tai Chi.

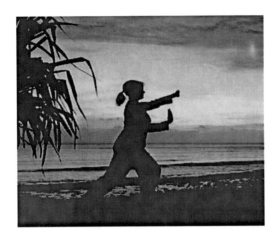

When Sun died, his daughter continued to teach the form in the same way as his father.

Basic Steps of Tai Chi for beginners

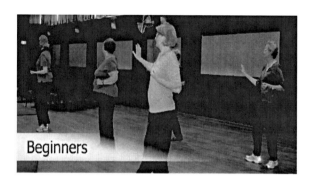

Beginners

Tai Chi is an ancient Chinese martial art form and is called the meditation in motion. The flowing movement of Tai Chi relieves stress and induces relaxation and creates a conscious awareness of the present moment.

Tai Chi reduces stress, depression and anxiety and improves your balance and coordination, reduces blood pressure, promotes sleep and has a lot of other benefits.

Tai Chi is a gentle and low impact exercise, so it suits any person with any level of physical fitness. The following are a few basic steps for beginners:

1. **Warm up-** Warming up the body is important for facilitating the movements of Tai Chi. Warm up Tai Chi exercises will open your body, helps promote a relaxed attitude in you and encourages your well being.

One of the basic warm up exercise in Tai Chi is loosening the waist. Stand on your feet parallel and at a hip width distance. Relax your arms at your sides, rotate your hips to the right side and then left. You have to move your arms along with the body movement. When your body has warmed up, incorporate your neck, shoulders and spine while rotating. Your movements have to be smooth and fluid.

2. **Windmill exercise-** This is one of basic movements in Tai Chi which promotes flexibility and opens your spine.

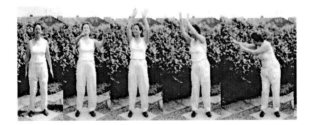

Stand with your feet parallel and slightly wider than shoulder-width distance apart. Relax your shoulders and let your arms hang loosely. Bring your hands in front of your body, point your fingers down towards the floor. Now inhale and raise the arms towards the body center and over your head, with fingers pointing up.

Now stretch towards the ceiling and arch your spine backwards a little. Now exhale and bend forwards, move your hands down towards the centre of your body. Bend forward from the hip joint, allowing your arms to hang in front of your body. Now inhale and return to your original position.

3. **Knee roll-** Knee roll will enhance the mobility in your spine and knees and will help in improving your balance. Stand with your feet a few inches apart and bend your knees slightly.

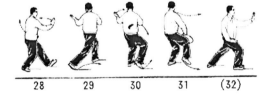

| 28 | 29 | 30 | 31 | (32) |

Keep your hands on your knees with fingers pointing to each other. Rotate your knees in a circle, roll from left, right and front like you are tracing a big circle on the floor with the knees. Perform circles in clockwise and anti-clockwise directions.

4. **Hand exercises-** Tai Chi hand exercises will open your hands; it promotes the flexibility in your arms, fingers and shoulders. Stand with feet at a shoulder width distance apart. Raise your arms straight out in front of you, parallel to the floor at shoulder height. Stretch your hands as much as you can and rotate your wrist in clockwise and anti-clockwise direction.

5. **Closing position-** Tai closing position is performed at the end of the practice to balance your energy and promote relaxation. Stand with your feet apart at a distance of hip apart. Relax your shoulders keep your hands in a cupped position with palms facing up and rest them in front of your pelvis. Now with closed eyes inhale and imagine you are pulling energy up and bring th hands to the centre of your body to your chest. Exhale and rotate your hands so that

your palms face down. You must imagine your energy pushing down as you move your hands towards the floor.

Do these exercises several times.

How to Do Tai Chi

Tai Chi is an ancient Chinese internal or soft martial art which is often practiced for health and spiritual benefits. It is a gentle and slow paced form. Tai Chi has a lot of benefits which increases strength, flexibility and mental concentration. If you are a beginner in Tai Chi then there are 4 forms you must follow 4 parts:

1. Breathing, form and style
2. Mastering the moves
3. Finding the right class
4. Becoming a pro

Breathing, form and style

You must warm up with proper breathing. You have to focus your chi, tap into yourself to find your potential and start with proper breathing.

- Position your feet at shoulder width distance
- Keep your hands on the abdomen, 5 cm below your navel and push in lightly.
- Breathe through your nose slowly in and out. Feel your abdomen move while breathing.

You have to concentrate on all the parts of your body while you are breathing. Now start relaxing each part of your body one at a time. Begin from your feet and go up. You will realize that you are holding tension after a while. You'll find you were holding tension without even realizing it.

Rooting is a concept of Tai Chi. Imagine you are a part of the ground and focus on your balance. When doing Tai Chi, your limbs will sway like branches in the wind, rooted to the ground. This does not imply that your legs are stiff. You have to imagine the roots under you, a part of you, allowing you for freedom or motion because you cannot fall, as you are a part of the natural world.

Different frames

1. *Small frame*- these forms are not very expansive. The movements are small and has less extension. It focuses on the internal energy to bring the right movements and transition.

2. *Large frame-* It involves low and high stances, postures which are dramatic and arm swinging. It concentrates on the right positioning and alignment of the body and develop energy.

3. *Medium frame-* This lies in between the two styles.

You have to experiment with different styles. All the styles are good, but it is good if you experiment. The Chen style is difficult for beginners, it is very slow than being explosive. The Yang style is popular, it uses large frame movements. The Wu style movements are microscopic. This style is easy to do but is hard to master. It focuses a lot on the energy flow and inner pressured movements. The movement are slow and deliberate.

Mastering Tai Chi Moves

The art of Tai Chi is improving the flow of Chi, the traditional Chinese life energy. Tai Chi improves many medical conditions physically and mentally. It is a low impact form so can be safely practiced by senior citizens too.

Tai Chi is attunement with the nature; it is more about the nature within us. So apart from providing health benefits and relieving stress, Tai Chi also means tapping into your inner self.

Tai Chi is not just about moving your hands slowly in front of you. Every movement in Tai Chi has a purpose and flow. It is easy to learn and retain a move when you know its purpose.

Tai chi is about the internal flow of energy. You have to examine the flow of energy and the body mechanics. Observe whether your body is compresses and storing energy or it opens and releasing the energy.

Class Tai Chi Moves

1. Commencement move- All most all the tai chi forms begin with this move. There are 4 major tai chi energies are found in this move, which preps the practitioner for the remaining of the form.

2. Single Whip- This is another well known Tai Chi move. In this move, one hand stays in the beak hand position. Four fingers lightly touch your thumb and your palm faces down. Arms are at shoulder height and spread like loose wings.

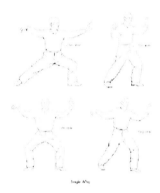

3. White Crane Spreads Wings- In this your weight must always bear on one leg and your feet has to be on the ground. You have to shift back and forth and test your balance. Keep your arms opposite, one

arm has to move fast and on different planes and the other has to be slow and deliberate.

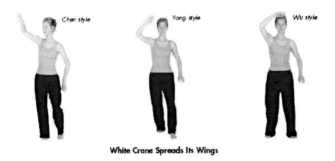

White Crane Spreads Its Wings

4. Pouring- Stand with feet apart on the floor at shoulder width apart, then pour your weight onto one leg and hold, after a few breathe in and outs you have to slowly pour your weight onto the other leg and hold. Clear your mind and be aware of your balance.

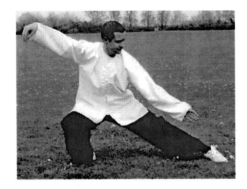

5. Snake creeps down- This move is a little different from other Tai Chi styles. You have to move from a standing posture to a deep lunge with grace.

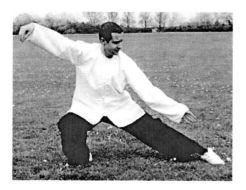

When you have moved, test your balance by moving your arms in different planes and speeds.

Find the right Tai Chi Class

There are many styles of Tai Chi and each of it has a special focus on health and martial arts. There are over 100 positions and movements in Tai Chi which you can learn. These movements carry the names of the animals and the nature.

Any person can do Tai Chi, it concentrates on the strength, providing a chance to master the art irrespective of the person's strength or age.

As you are a beginner, you have to find the right teacher, there are no degrees and credentials in teaching Tai Chi. The key factor is the compatibility in your learning style with the teaching style of your teacher.

As there is not universal accreditation system for Tai Chi teachers, it makes it difficult for a beginner to judge the teacher's suitability. You have to choose a teacher who can guide you well and answers all your questions. You can also learn from another advanced student as you are still a beginner.

Becoming a professional

You have to keep practicing Tai Chi if you want to improve your tai chi skills. Practice it at least once in a day. Practicing 2 times a week is the minimum amount to learn the most effectively and feel its benefits.

You have to develop a routine so that it is easy to remember and you feel good during the day. The benefits you derive from practicing Tai Chi depends on developing a routine, how you practice and the consistency of the practice. Set at least 15 minutes everyday to practice Tai Chi. You can practice it indoors or outdoors, solo or with friends as a group.

You have to practice at least 12 weeks so that you will start noticing the benefits. But continue practicing even after 3 months to continue enjoying the benefits and improve your skill.

How Tai Chi Helps Find Peace and Serenity

Tai Chi is a martial arts form. The term martial arts evokes the images of fighting an violence, but it has a lot of benefits and can be practices by persons of any age and any strength.

Many of Tai Chi practitioners have adopted Tai Chi as not only a form of martial arts but its techniques for relieving stress and inducing relaxation. Though it has been found in China, it has spread to different parts of the world and is practiced mainly to reduce stress and anxiety and to help the individuals find serenity and inner peace.

Many people are experiencing stress and anxiety now-a-days because of the change in lifestyle and work and other things. This stress is causing depression, alcoholism, substance abuse etc. Sometimes the problem becomes so severe that the person can no longer carry out normal functions of every day. This affects the individual a lot.

Stress and anxiety can be treated and addresses in many ways with therapeutic options. They can be treated at therapy centers, psychiatric centers etc. Here the patient is provided counseling, coaching and lifestyle changes. In severe cases, medication is also advised.

Other effective ways of managing stress is by practicing Tai Chi, which is an ancient Chinese martial arts form which helps promote health and longevity. Tai Chi can be practiced solo at home or can be practiced as a group in parks and outdoors. It promoted relaxation. The deliberate and slow movements of the hands, arms, torso, legs and feet promote flexibility too. The movements helps increase circulation and treat many ailments. However, the main effect it creates is reducing stress and providing relaxation.

Whether you perform it as a group or solo, it will reduce your anxiety, drive away all your negative thoughts and worries and helps you connect with your inner self and find serenity.

Feelings are subjective and relative so you will start feeling confidence and peace on an off from the first few months you start learning Tai Chi. Tai Chi study has hills and valleys in it. Sometimes you will feel like you are on the top of the world and then you make a breakthrough. But during the process your will know where you can grow your skills.

As you learn and practice Tai Chi every day, you will feel closer to your goals, you will find where you need to progress and improve your skills. As you progress you will see the opportunities to learn and you have to embrace these opportunities as you are beginner and help yourself in finding serenity and inner peace.

Benefits of Tai Chi

Tai Chi has a lot of physical and psychological benefits. A few are:

Physical benefits

1. Improves strength and balance- Tai chi reduces the fear of falling and the risk of falling, hence it can be safely practiced by senior citizens too. The slow and coordinated movements of each form improve the strength of the person practicing it and also the balance, which are usually low in old people.

2. Reduces pain- People suffering from arthritis and other painful conditions can practice tai chi and research shows that those who participated in these sessions have lesser joint pain and stiffness.

3. Improves immunity- Tai Chi helps improve immunity and so you will fall less prone to common cold, coughs and other ailments.

4. For diabetes- Tai Chi can improve blood glucose levels and the immune system response in patients suffering from type II Diabetes.

5. Improves functions- Tai Chi can improve cardiovascular, lymphatic, respiratory and digestive system functions.

6. Range of motion- It improves your range of motion in the joints and their flexibility.

7. Leg strength- As Tai Chi involves many movements of the leg, the stance; the movements all improve the strength in the legs.

8. It increases your energy including sexual vitality and fertility.

Psychological benefits

1. Improves sleep- Tai Chi impacts your sleep. It improves the sleep quality and length.

2. Helps fight stress- Tai Chi enhances the overall psychological well being. It improves your mood which in turn helps fight stress.

3. It reduces depression, anxiety and tension

4. It will improve your breath control and meditation capacity. It also improves your cognitive brain functions.

CPSIA information can be obtained at www.ICGtesting.com
Printed in the USA
LVOW10s0051110816

499914LV00031B/346/P